Wiggle your toes and touch your nose.
Now, can you guess the yoga pose?

I am a riddle. I am a rhyme.
I stretch the body and tickle the mind.

What am I?

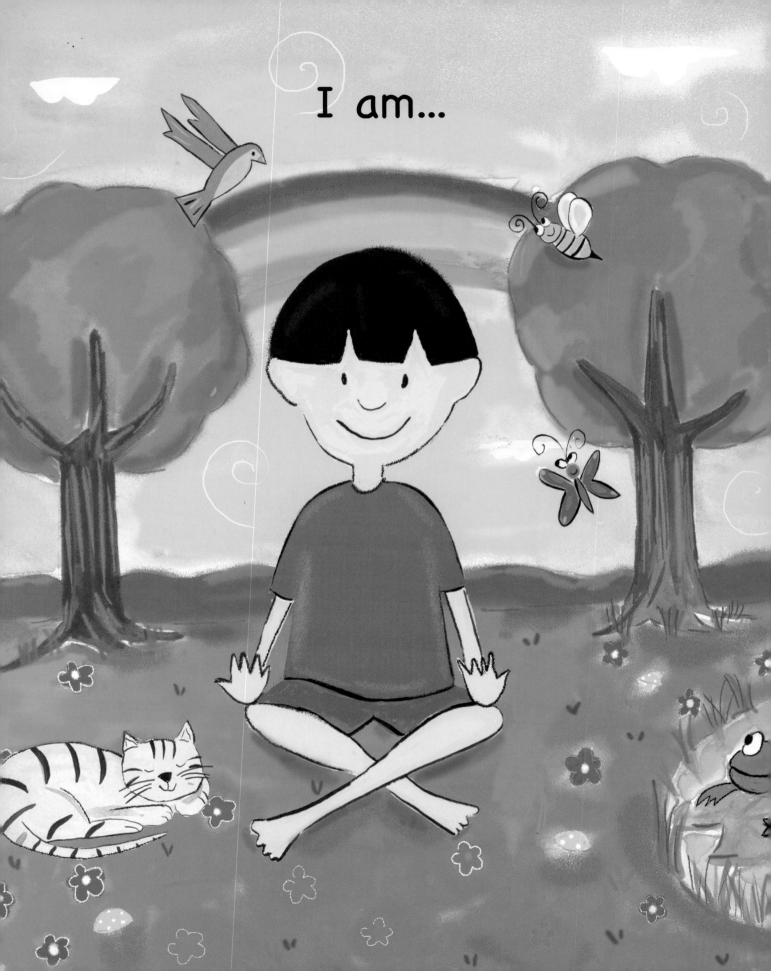

I am...

THE
YOGA GAME

by **Kathy Beliveau**   illustrated by **Farida Zaman**

SIMPLY READ BOOKS

Things to remember
while playing The Yoga Game!

It is better to wait up to two hours after eating before practicing yoga.

Yoga is normally practiced in comfortable clothes and barefoot to prevent slipping. (A sticky mat is useful but not essential.)

Yoga is not about competition. Never push yourself or force the postures.

In yoga, keep your body relaxed and your breathing slow and steady.

Ready?

It's time to play!

I flit and flutter everywhere,
happy, free, as light as air.
With silent grace,
I land on things,
and sunlight dances on my wings.

What am I?

I am a butterfly!

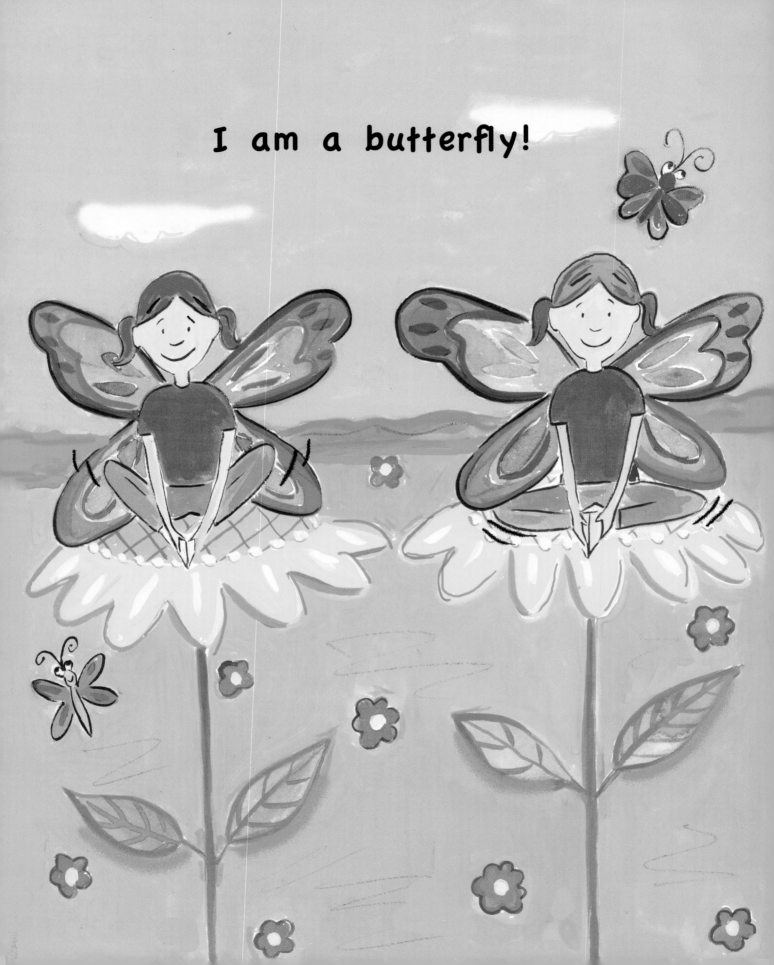

Softer than a breath, that's me.
I'm known to be bumbly.
A ball of black and yellow fuzz,
my song is like a low, deep buzzzz.

What am I?

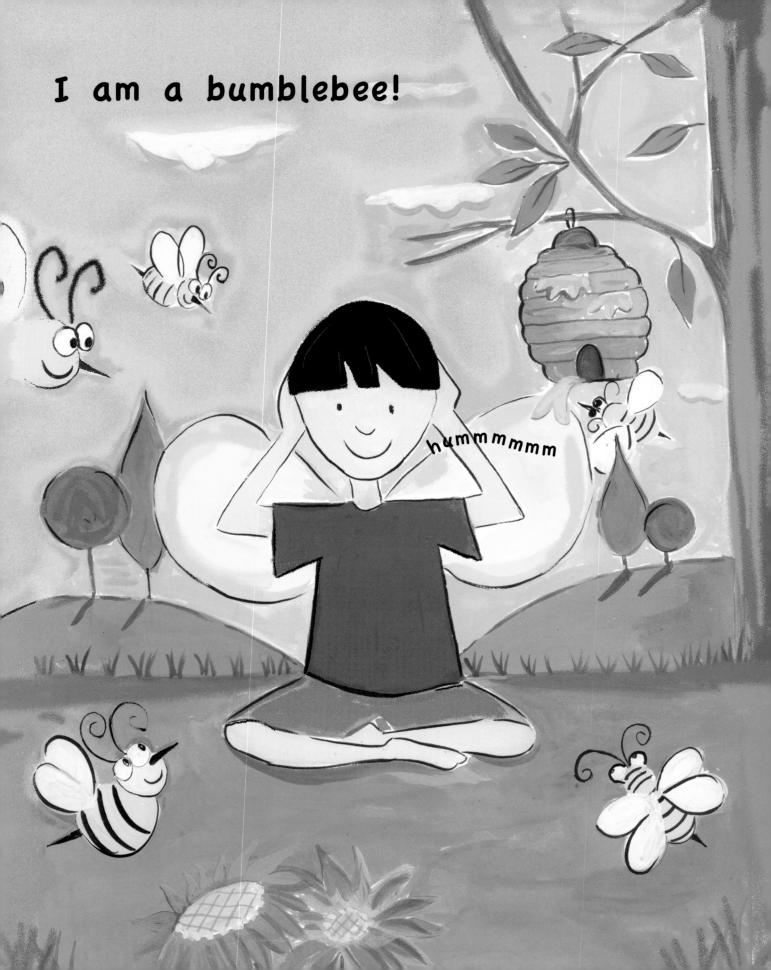

One foot stands planted on the ground,
and in my mind I send roots down.
Balancing, my arms stretch high,
like branches reaching to the sky.

What am I?

I am a tree!

I love a place that's
    warm and nice,
to rest my paws
    and dream of mice.
Where in between
    my nap and snack,
there's time to arch
    and stretch my back.

What am I?

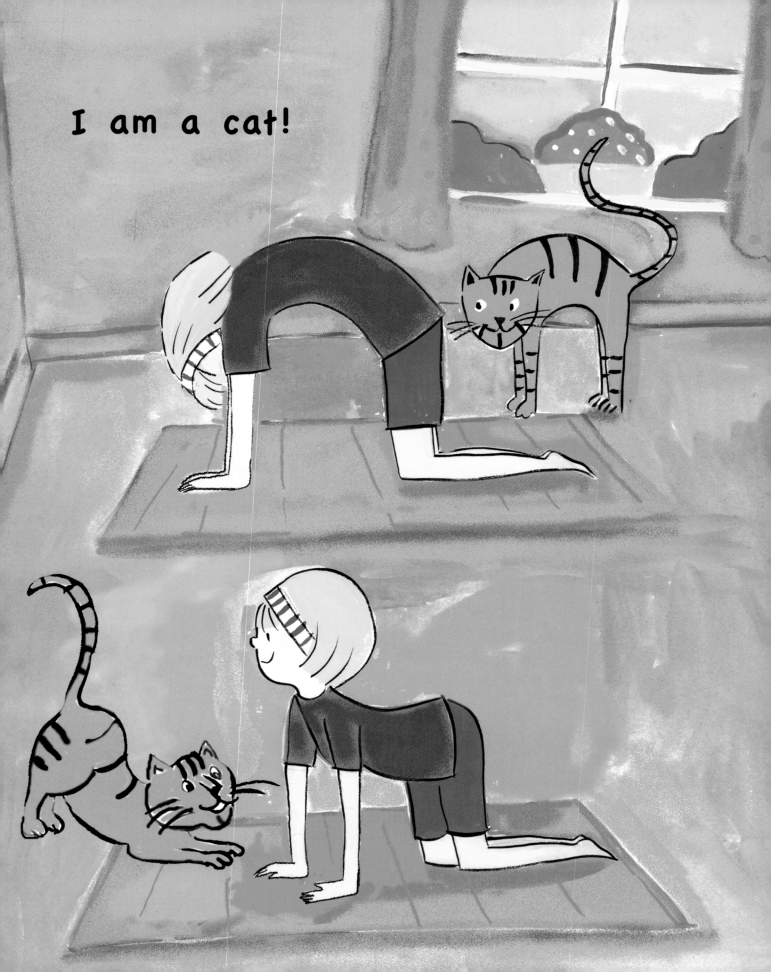

I am a cat!

I can reach way up high
and paint my magic in the sky.
Radiant colours everywhere,
see them balance in the air.

What am I?

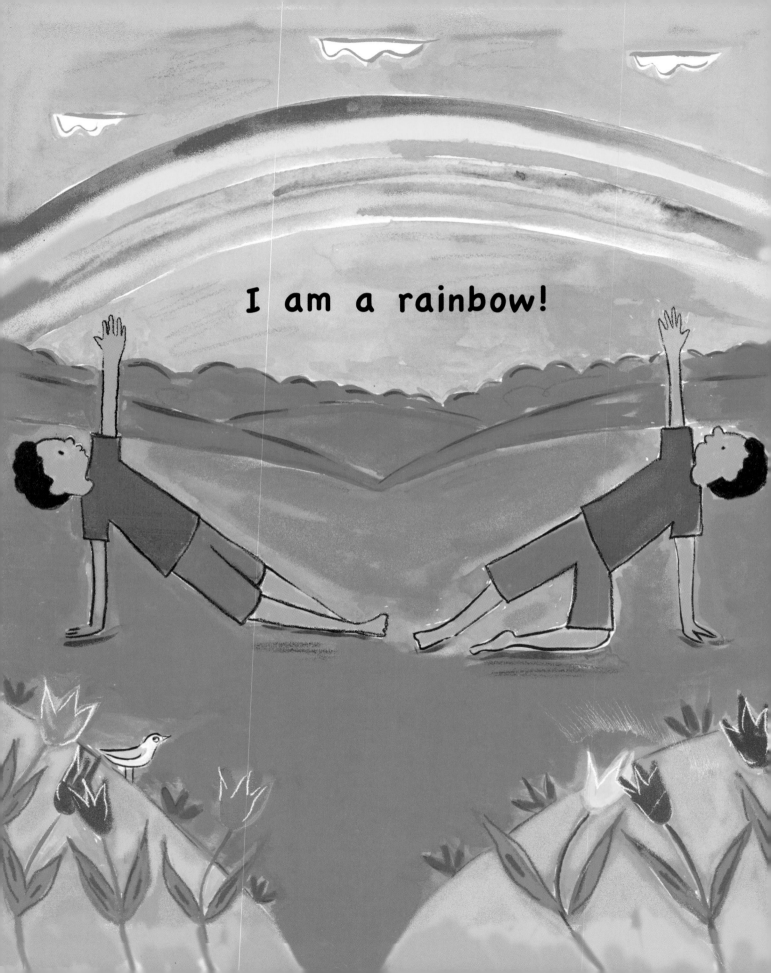

I am a rainbow!

No arms or legs
     to help me climb,
I slither and slide
     along my spine.
Some say I have
a dangerous kiss.
Beware of me.
When I stretch,
     I hissss.

What am I?

I am a cobra!

I am grey. I am small.
My back is rounded
like a ball.

I nibble cheese
and things like that,
then scamper past
and tease the cat.

What am I?

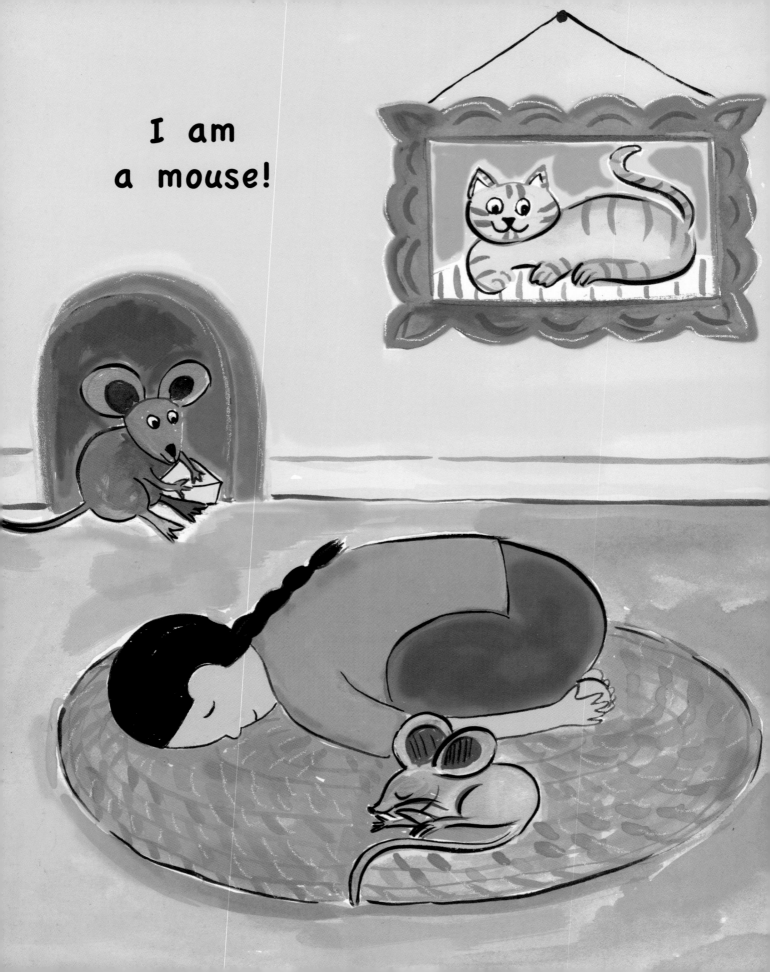

I am much bigger than a hill.
I stand strong. I stand still.
Though wind and snow cover my face
I stand majestic in my place.

What am I?

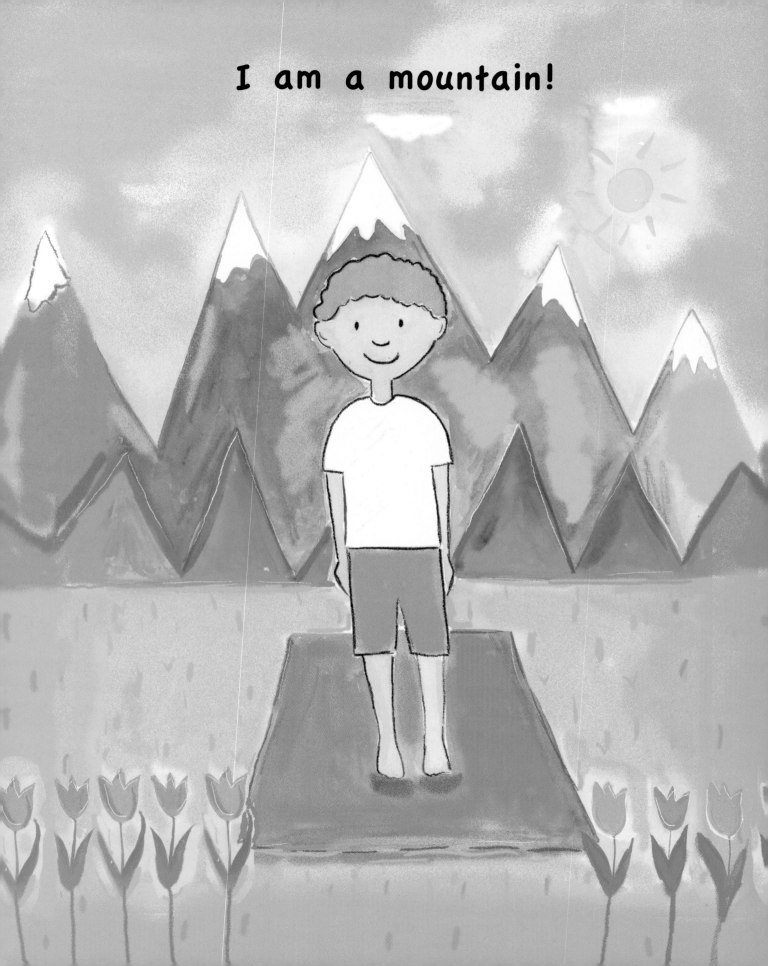

I am a mountain!

I soar above the land and sea
or sit upon a giant tree.
Perching poised with piercing eyes,
I silently search sea and skies.

What am I?

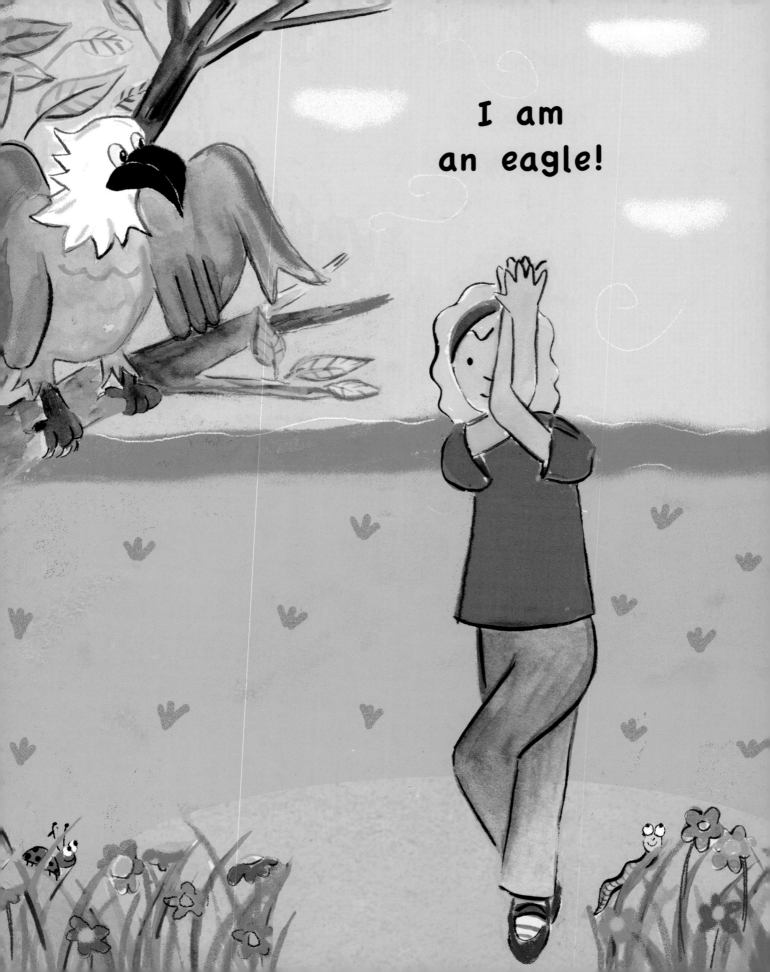

They call me King,
though I have
no crown.
But I can make
a mighty sound!

I crouch down low
on the jungle floor.
And then I leap
and pounce and ROAR!

What am I?

I am a lion!

I burst up through the warm blue sea.
Then dive down low and splash with glee.
I click and cluck and whistle sound.
My laughter bubbles all around.

What am I?

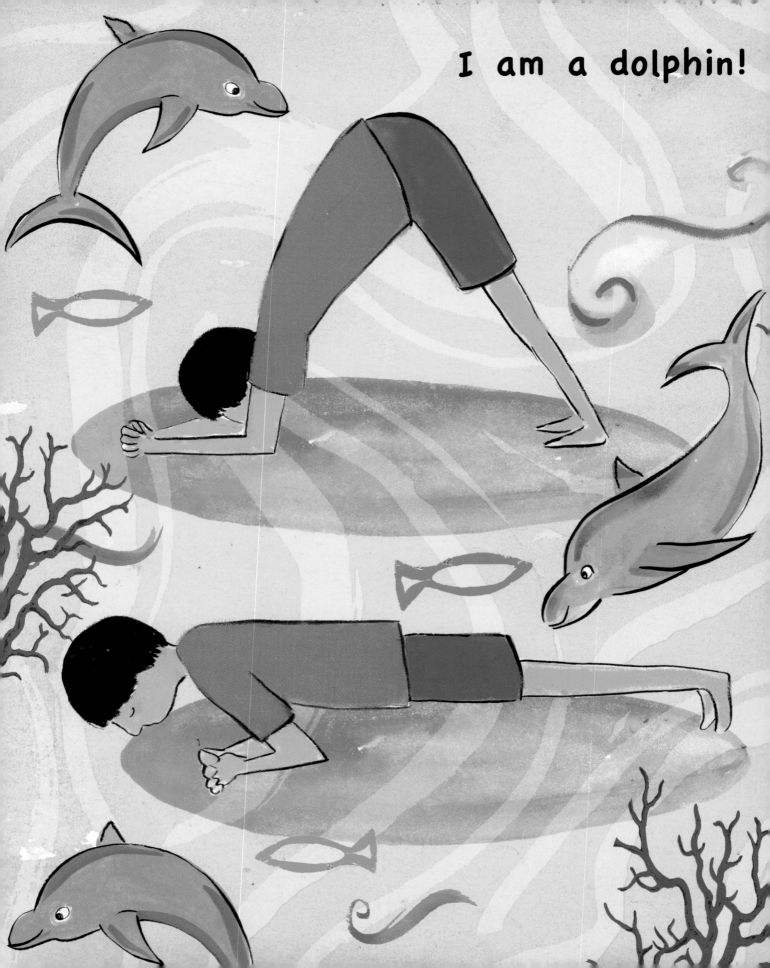

I am a dolphin!

I stretch my arms
    and legs out wide.
I hold my head
    with grace and pride.
I glow and twinkle
    and shine so bright.
It feels good to
    share my light.

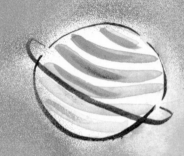

What am I?

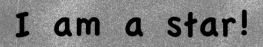

I am a star!

The squishy mud of lakes and ponds
inspires me to sing my songs.
I croak, I swim, I hop about.
I squat and stick my tongue way out.

What am I?

I am a frog!

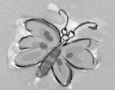

I have a hump
    upon my back.
It is my secret
    water sack.

I come from an exotic land,
of scorching sun and desert sand.

What am I?

I am a camel!

Slow and steady wins the race.
I do not like a hectic pace.
A simple shell is all I own,
to go within, to be at home.

What am I?

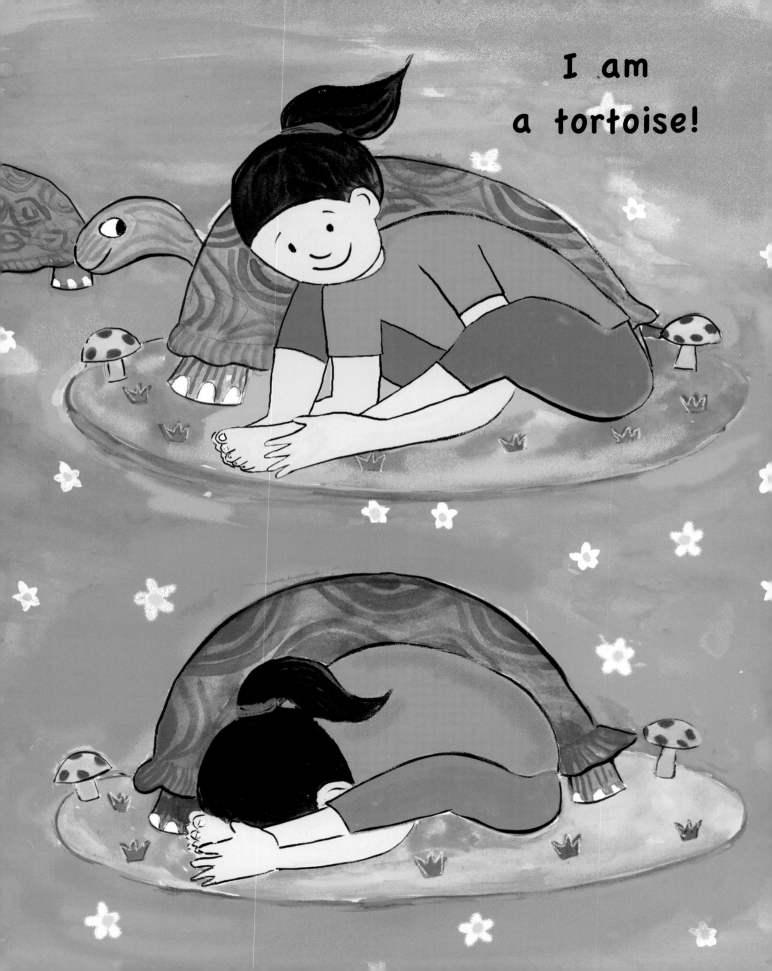

I am
a tortoise!

I breathe the air,
the air breathes me.
I am the land. I am the sea.
I am a cloud that drifts above.
I am special.
I am love.

What am I?

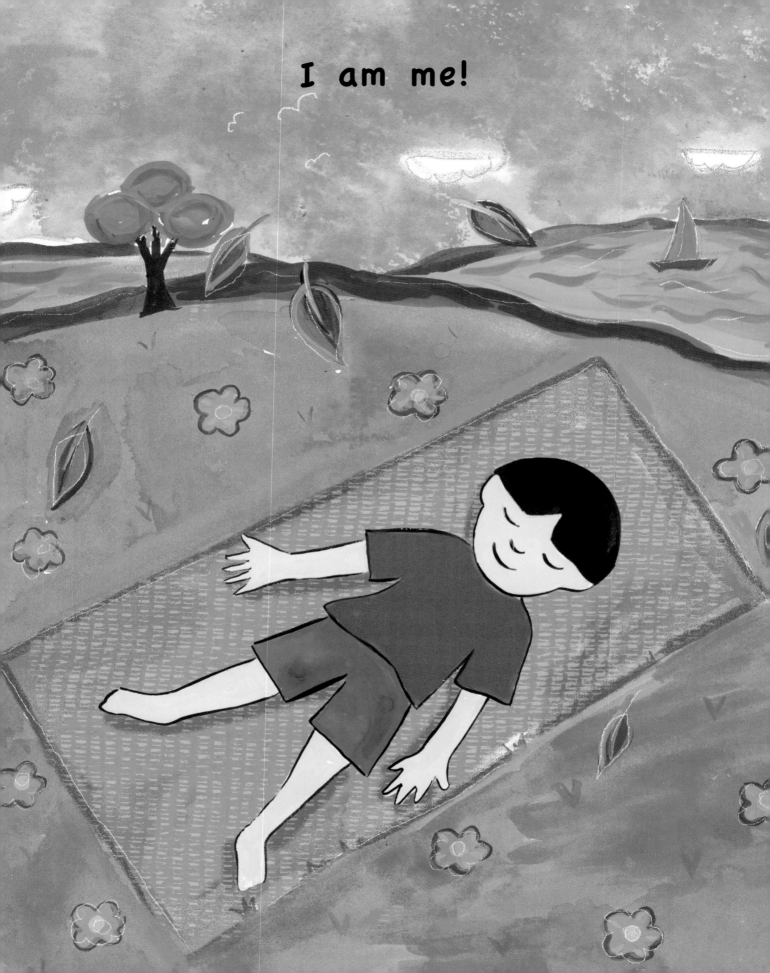

Namaste!

What is yoga?

Yoga is an ancient practice originating in India over 5,000 years ago.

The word yoga comes from Sanskrit and means to unite or bring together. The practice of yoga helps to bring together body, mind and spirit.

Hatha Yoga is the physical practice of asana or postures, along with breathing practices and meditation.

Yoga is much more than an exercise. Yoga is a way of life that includes proper exercise, breathing, diet, relaxation and positive thought. It is a journey of self-discovery.

* * * * * * *

"Smile with the flower and the green grass. Play with the butterflies, birds and deer. Shake hands with the shrubs, ferns and twigs of trees. Talk to the rainbow, wind, stars and the sun. Converse with the running brooks and the waves of the sea. Speak with the walking-stick. Develop friendships with all your neighbors, dogs, cats, cows, human beings, trees, flowers, etc. Then you will have a wide, perfect, rich, full life. You will realize oneness or unity of life. This can be hardly described in words. You will have to feel this yourself."

—Swami Sivananda

About the Author

Kathy Beliveau has always loved nature, writing and pretty much anything that feeds the soul. Kathy's relationship with yoga began as a preteen and has continued to develop over the years. She has studied Children's Yoga and is a Certified Yoga Instructor. As well, Kathy writes for children and adults and has enjoyed recognition in contests and literary magazines. Her stories have entertained primary grades and preschools; they have been performed by a storybook theatre and used by special needs programs. In a light and playful style, her stories connect kids with nature; they connect people to the planet; and they connect body, mind and spirit. Kathy lives on Vancouver Island, BC, with her husband, youngest daughter and several cats. www.kathybeliveau.ca

About the Illustrator

Farida Zaman has a passion for art and design. In her 20 years as a freelance illustrator, Farida has worked in many countries across the world, bringing style, colour and joy to many. A graduate of the Chelsea College of Art and the Wimbledon School of Art, both in London, England, she has illustrated numerous children's books, and her work has been used in advertising, packaging, greeting cards, newspapers and magazines throughout Britain, Canada, and the United States. Farida Zaman and her husband have two children and live in Toronto, Ontario. www.faridazaman.com

For all my teachers, for my "encouragers"
and for my enchanting daughters,
Kalila, Teesha and Maya.
Thank you for shining so bright
and sharing your light. Namaste.

KB

To Layla and Gibran,
Kiyan and Kira.
With lots of love
and hugs always.

FZ

Published in 2012 by Simply Read Books www.simplyreadbooks.com
Text © 2012 Kathy Beliveau
Illustrations © 2012 Farida Zaman

Library and Archives Canada Cataloguing in Publication

Beliveau, Kathy, 1962-
        The yoga game / written by Kathy Beliveau ; illustrated by Farida Zaman.

ISBN 978-1-897476-72-7

1. Hatha yoga--Juvenile literature.
I. Zaman, Farida II. Title.

RA781.7.B44 2012   j613.7'046   C2011-907046-4

We gratefully acknowledge for their financial support of our publishing program the Canada Council for the Arts, the BC Arts Council, and the Government of Canada through the Canada Book Fund (CBF).

Manufactured in Singapore

10 9 8 7 6 5 4 3 2 1